# Healthy Data

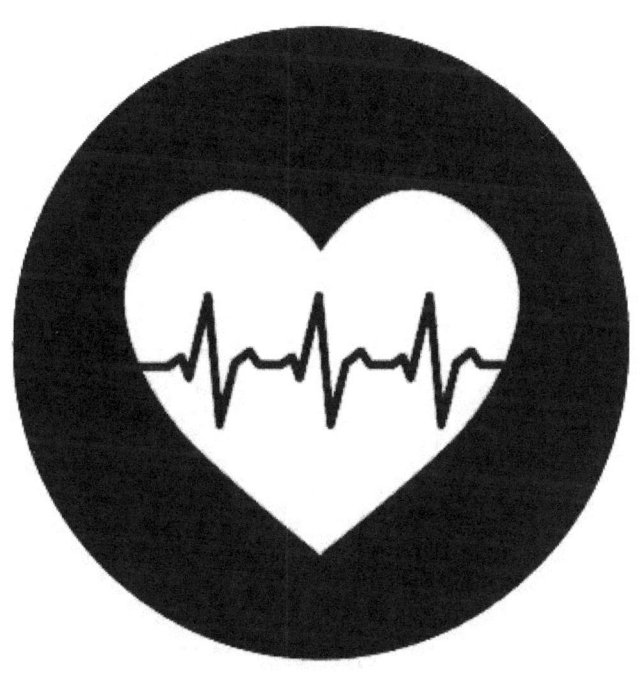

# Personal Information

Name

Birthday

Blood type

My address

Weight

Height

# With our Healthy Data

You Could maintain your health
while still  healthy
Is  the most Beatiful moment in your life

Benefits Of Self Balancing Food

Ella Woo

**ISBN-13:**
**978-1547141104**

**ISBN-10:**
**1547141107**

# Nutrition Information

Serving size: ............... Scoop  (...................grams)
Serving per container: .................

---

**Amount per serving**
**Total Calories** ........kg.     Calories from fat ...kg. Calories

---

## Percent Daily Values

| | | |
|---|---|---|
| **Total fat** | ......g | .....% |
| Saturated | ......g | .....% |
| **Cholesterol** | ......mg | .....% |
| **Protein** | ......g | |
| **Total carbohydrate** | ......g | ......% |
| Dietary fiber | ......g | ......% |
| Sugar | ......g | |
| **Sodium** (Na) | ......mg | .......% |

---

## Percent Daily Values

| | | | |
|---|---|---|---|
| Vitamin A | ..........% | Vitamin B1 | ..........% |
| Vitamin B2 | ..........% | Calcium (Ca) | ..........% |
| Iron (Fe) | ..........% | | |

My Body, Date........./.......

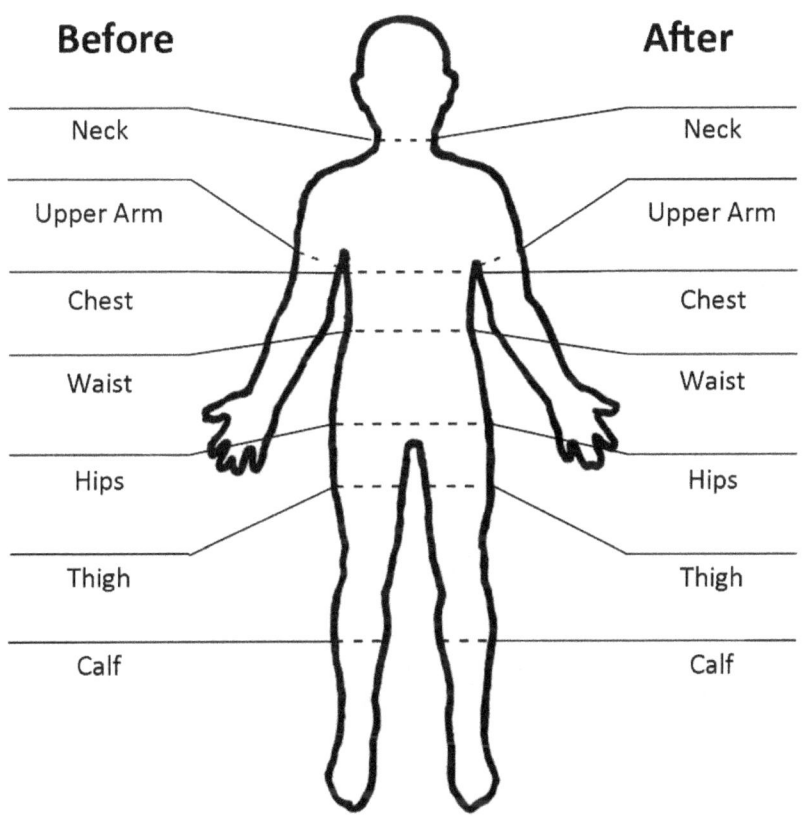

**Before**

Neck

Upper Arm

Chest

Waist

Hips

Thigh

Calf

**After**

Neck

Upper Arm

Chest

Waist

Hips

Thigh

Calf

No........ Date........../..........

| | M | T | W | TH | F | S | S |
|---|---|---|---|---|---|---|---|
| Drink Wather | | | | | | | |
| Breakfast | | | | | | | |
| Lunch | | | | | | | |
| Diner | | | | | | | |
| **Sleep** | | | | | | | |
| **Active** | | | | | | | |
| Snack 1 | | | | | | | |
| **Snack 2** | | | | | | | |
| **Snack 3** | | | | | | | |
| **Party** | | | | | | | |

## Food list

| Vegetables | Grain | Meat |
|---|---|---|
| ☐ Almond | ☐ Adzuki Beans | ☐ Fish |
| ☐ Cabbage | ☐ Barley | ☐ Goat |
| ☐ Carrot | ☐ Black Bean | ☐ Pork |
| ☐ Boccoli | ☐ Brown Rice | ☐ Beef |
| ☐ Garlic | ☐ Buckwheat | ☐ Lamb |
| ☐ Licorice | ☐ Job'sTears, Adlay | ☐ Chicken |
| ☐ Onion | ☐ Millet | ☐ _____ |
| ☐ Spinach | ☐ Mung Beans | ☐ _____ |
| ☐ Sweet potato | ☐ Sesame | ☐ _____ |
| ☐ Tomato | ☐ Sorghum | |
| ☐ _____ | ☐ _____ | |
| ☐ _____ | ☐ _____ | |
| ☐ _____ | ☐ _____ | |

Note:..................................................................................................
..................................................................................................

No........ Date........../..........

| | M | T | W | TH | F | S | S |
|---|---|---|---|---|---|---|---|
| Drink Wather | | | | | | | |
| Breakfast | | | | | | | |
| Lunch | | | | | | | |
| Diner | | | | | | | |
| **Sleep** | | | | | | | |
| **Active** | | | | | | | |
| Snack 1 | | | | | | | |
| **Snack 2** | | | | | | | |
| **Snack 3** | | | | | | | |
| **Party** | | | | | | | |

## Food List

| Vegetables | Grain | Meat |
|---|---|---|
| ☐ Almond | ☐ Adzuki Beans | ☐ Fish |
| ☐ Cabbage | ☐ Barley | ☐ Goat |
| ☐ Carrot | ☐ Black Bean | ☐ Pork |
| ☐ Boccoli | ☐ Brown Rice | ☐ Beef |
| ☐ Garlic | ☐ Buckwheat | ☐ Lamb |
| ☐ Licorice | ☐ Job'sTears, Adlay | ☐ Chicken |
| ☐ Onion | ☐ Millet | ☐ _____ |
| ☐ Spinach | ☐ Mung Beans | ☐ _____ |
| ☐ Sweet potato | ☐ Sesame | ☐ _____ |
| ☐ Tomato | ☐ Sorghum | |
| ☐ _____ | ☐ _____ | |
| ☐ _____ | ☐ _____ | |
| ☐ _____ | ☐ _____ | |

Note:....................................................................................................
....................................................................................................

No........ Date........../..........

| | M | T | W | TH | F | S | S |
|---|---|---|---|---|---|---|---|
| Drink Wather | | | | | | | |
| Breakfast | | | | | | | |
| Lunch | | | | | | | |
| Diner | | | | | | | |
| **Sleep** | | | | | | | |
| **Active** | | | | | | | |
| Snack 1 | | | | | | | |
| **Snack 2** | | | | | | | |
| **Snack 3** | | | | | | | |
| **Party** | | | | | | | |

## Food list

| Vegetables | Grain | Meat |
|---|---|---|
| ☐ Almond | ☐ Adzuki Beans | ☐ Fish |
| ☐ Cabbage | ☐ Barley | ☐ Goat |
| ☐ Carrot | ☐ Black Bean | ☐ Pork |
| ☐ Boccoli | ☐ Brown Rice | ☐ Beef |
| ☐ Garlic | ☐ Buckwheat | ☐ Lamb |
| ☐ Licorice | ☐ Job'sTears, Adlay | ☐ Chicken |
| ☐ Onion | ☐ Millet | ☐ _____ |
| ☐ Spinach | ☐ Mung Beans | ☐ _____ |
| ☐ Sweet potato | ☐ Sesame | ☐ _____ |
| ☐ Tomato | ☐ Sorghum | |
| ☐ _____ | ☐ _____ | |
| ☐ _____ | ☐ _____ | |
| ☐ _____ | ☐ _____ | |

Note:.......................................................................................................
................................................................................................................

No........ Date........../..........

| | M | T | W | TH | F | S | S |
|---|---|---|---|---|---|---|---|
| Drink Wather | | | | | | | |
| Breakfast | | | | | | | |
| Lunch | | | | | | | |
| Diner | | | | | | | |
| **Sleep** | | | | | | | |
| **Active** | | | | | | | |
| Snack 1 | | | | | | | |
| **Snack 2** | | | | | | | |
| **Snack 3** | | | | | | | |
| **Party** | | | | | | | |

## Food list

| Vegetables | Grain | Meat |
|---|---|---|
| ☐ Almond | ☐ Adzuki Beans | ☐ Fish |
| ☐ Cabbage | ☐ Barley | ☐ Goat |
| ☐ Carrot | ☐ Black Bean | ☐ Pork |
| ☐ Boccoli | ☐ Brown Rice | ☐ Beef |
| ☐ Garlic | ☐ Buckwheat | ☐ Lamb |
| ☐ Licorice | ☐ Job'sTears, Adlay | ☐ Chicken |
| ☐ Onion | ☐ Millet | ☐ _____ |
| ☐ Spinach | ☐ Mung Beans | ☐ _____ |
| ☐ Sweet potato | ☐ Sesame | ☐ _____ |
| ☐ Tomato | ☐ Sorghum | |
| ☐ _____ | ☐ _____ | |
| ☐ _____ | ☐ _____ | |
| ☐ _____ | ☐ _____ | |

Note:..........................................................................................
..........................................................................................
..........................................................................................

No........ Date........../..........

| | M | T | W | TH | F | S | S |
|---|---|---|---|---|---|---|---|
| Drink Wather | | | | | | | |
| Breakfast | | | | | | | |
| Lunch | | | | | | | |
| Diner | | | | | | | |
| **Sleep** | | | | | | | |
| **Active** | | | | | | | |
| Snack 1 | | | | | | | |
| **Snack 2** | | | | | | | |
| **Snack 3** | | | | | | | |
| **Party** | | | | | | | |

## Food list

| Vegetables | Grain | Meat |
|---|---|---|
| ☐ Almond | ☐ Adzuki Beans | ☐ Fish |
| ☐ Cabbage | ☐ Barley | ☐ Goat |
| ☐ Carrot | ☐ Black Bean | ☐ Pork |
| ☐ Boccoli | ☐ Brown Rice | ☐ Beef |
| ☐ Garlic | ☐ Buckwheat | ☐ Lamb |
| ☐ Licorice | ☐ Job'sTears, Adlay | ☐ Chicken |
| ☐ Onion | ☐ Millet | ☐ _____ |
| ☐ Spinach | ☐ Mung Beans | ☐ _____ |
| ☐ Sweet potato | ☐ Sesame | ☐ _____ |
| ☐ Tomato | ☐ Sorghum | |
| ☐ _____ | ☐ _____ | |
| ☐ _____ | ☐ _____ | |
| ☐ _____ | ☐ _____ | |

Note:...........................................................................................
.............................................................................................
.............................................................................................

No........ Date........../..........

| | M | T | W | TH | F | S | S |
|---|---|---|---|---|---|---|---|
| Drink Wather | | | | | | | |
| Breakfast | | | | | | | |
| Lunch | | | | | | | |
| Diner | | | | | | | |
| **Sleep** | | | | | | | |
| **Active** | | | | | | | |
| Snack 1 | | | | | | | |
| **Snack 2** | | | | | | | |
| **Snack 3** | | | | | | | |
| **Party** | | | | | | | |

## Food list

| Vegetables | Grain | Meat |
|---|---|---|
| ☐ Almond | ☐ Adzuki Beans | ☐ Fish |
| ☐ Cabbage | ☐ Barley | ☐ Goat |
| ☐ Carrot | ☐ Black Bean | ☐ Pork |
| ☐ Boccoli | ☐ Brown Rice | ☐ Beef |
| ☐ Garlic | ☐ Buckwheat | ☐ Lamb |
| ☐ Licorice | ☐ Job'sTears, Adlay | ☐ Chicken |
| ☐ Onion | ☐ Millet | ☐ _____ |
| ☐ Spinach | ☐ Mung Beans | ☐ _____ |
| ☐ Sweet potato | ☐ Sesame | ☐ _____ |
| ☐ Tomato | ☐ Sorghum | |
| ☐ _____ | ☐ _____ | |
| ☐ _____ | ☐ _____ | |
| ☐ _____ | ☐ _____ | |

Note:.................................................................................
.................................................................................
.................................................................................

No........ Date........../..........

| | M | T | W | TH | F | S | S |
|---|---|---|---|---|---|---|---|
| Drink Wather | | | | | | | |
| Breakfast | | | | | | | |
| Lunch | | | | | | | |
| Diner | | | | | | | |
| **Sleep** | | | | | | | |
| **Active** | | | | | | | |
| Snack 1 | | | | | | | |
| **Snack 2** | | | | | | | |
| **Snack 3** | | | | | | | |
| **Party** | | | | | | | |

## Food list

| Vegetables | Grain | Meat |
|---|---|---|
| ☐ Almond | ☐ Adzuki Beans | ☐ Fish |
| ☐ Cabbage | ☐ Barley | ☐ Goat |
| ☐ Carrot | ☐ Black Bean | ☐ Pork |
| ☐ Boccoli | ☐ Brown Rice | ☐ Beef |
| ☐ Garlic | ☐ Buckwheat | ☐ Lamb |
| ☐ Licorice | ☐ Job'sTears, Adlay | ☐ Chicken |
| ☐ Onion | ☐ Millet | ☐ _____ |
| ☐ Spinach | ☐ Mung Beans | ☐ _____ |
| ☐ Sweet potato | ☐ Sesame | ☐ _____ |
| ☐ Tomato | ☐ Sorghum | |
| ☐ _____ | ☐ _____ | |
| ☐ _____ | ☐ _____ | |
| ☐ _____ | ☐ _____ | |

Note:...............................................................................................
.......................................................................................................
.......................................................................................................

No........ Date........../..........

| | M | T | W | TH | F | S | S |
|---|---|---|---|---|---|---|---|
| Drink Wather | | | | | | | |
| Breakfast | | | | | | | |
| Lunch | | | | | | | |
| Diner | | | | | | | |
| **Sleep** | | | | | | | |
| **Active** | | | | | | | |
| Snack 1 | | | | | | | |
| **Snack 2** | | | | | | | |
| **Snack 3** | | | | | | | |
| **Party** | | | | | | | |

## Food list

| Vegetables | Grain | Meat |
|---|---|---|
| ☐ Almond | ☐ Adzuki Beans | ☐ Fish |
| ☐ Cabbage | ☐ Barley | ☐ Goat |
| ☐ Carrot | ☐ Black Bean | ☐ Pork |
| ☐ Boccoli | ☐ Brown Rice | ☐ Beef |
| ☐ Garlic | ☐ Buckwheat | ☐ Lamb |
| ☐ Licorice | ☐ Job'sTears, Adlay | ☐ Chicken |
| ☐ Onion | ☐ Millet | ☐ _____ |
| ☐ Spinach | ☐ Mung Beans | ☐ _____ |
| ☐ Sweet potato | ☐ Sesame | ☐ _____ |
| ☐ Tomato | ☐ Sorghum | |
| ☐ _____ | ☐ _____ | |
| ☐ _____ | ☐ _____ | |
| ☐ _____ | ☐ _____ | |

Note:..................................................................................................
..................................................................................................
..................................................................................................

No........ Date........../..........

| | M | T | W | TH | F | S | S |
|---|---|---|---|---|---|---|---|
| Drink Wather | | | | | | | |
| Breakfast | | | | | | | |
| Lunch | | | | | | | |
| Diner | | | | | | | |
| **Sleep** | | | | | | | |
| **Active** | | | | | | | |
| Snack 1 | | | | | | | |
| **Snack 2** | | | | | | | |
| **Snack 3** | | | | | | | |
| **Party** | | | | | | | |

## Food list

| Vegetables | Grain | Meat |
|---|---|---|
| ☐ Almond | ☐ Adzuki Beans | ☐ Fish |
| ☐ Cabbage | ☐ Barley | ☐ Goat |
| ☐ Carrot | ☐ Black Bean | ☐ Pork |
| ☐ Boccoli | ☐ Brown Rice | ☐ Beef |
| ☐ Garlic | ☐ Buckwheat | ☐ Lamb |
| ☐ Licorice | ☐ Job'sTears, Adlay | ☐ Chicken |
| ☐ Onion | ☐ Millet | ☐ _____ |
| ☐ Spinach | ☐ Mung Beans | ☐ _____ |
| ☐ Sweet potato | ☐ Sesame | ☐ _____ |
| ☐ Tomato | ☐ Sorghum | |
| ☐ _____ | ☐ _____ | |
| ☐ _____ | ☐ _____ | |
| ☐ _____ | ☐ _____ | |

Note:.................................................................................................
.................................................................................................
.................................................................................................

No........ Date........../..........

| | M | T | W | TH | F | S | S |
|---|---|---|---|---|---|---|---|
| Drink Wather | | | | | | | |
| Breakfast | | | | | | | |
| Lunch | | | | | | | |
| Diner | | | | | | | |
| **Sleep** | | | | | | | |
| **Active** | | | | | | | |
| Snack 1 | | | | | | | |
| **Snack 2** | | | | | | | |
| **Snack 3** | | | | | | | |
| **Party** | | | | | | | |

## Food list

| Vegetables | Grain | Meat |
|---|---|---|
| ☐ Almond | ☐ Adzuki Beans | ☐ Fish |
| ☐ Cabbage | ☐ Barley | ☐ Goat |
| ☐ Carrot | ☐ Black Bean | ☐ Pork |
| ☐ Boccoli | ☐ Brown Rice | ☐ Beef |
| ☐ Garlic | ☐ Buckwheat | ☐ Lamb |
| ☐ Licorice | ☐ Job'sTears, Adlay | ☐ Chicken |
| ☐ Onion | ☐ Millet | ☐ _____ |
| ☐ Spinach | ☐ Mung Beans | ☐ _____ |
| ☐ Sweet potato | ☐ Sesame | ☐ _____ |
| ☐ Tomato | ☐ Sorghum | |
| ☐ _____ | ☐ _____ | |
| ☐ _____ | ☐ _____ | |
| ☐ _____ | ☐ _____ | |

Note:...........................................................................................
.......................................................................................................
.......................................................................................................

No........ Date........../..........

| | M | T | W | TH | F | S | S |
|---|---|---|---|---|---|---|---|
| Drink Wather | | | | | | | |
| Breakfast | | | | | | | |
| Lunch | | | | | | | |
| Diner | | | | | | | |
| Sleep | | | | | | | |
| Active | | | | | | | |
| Snack 1 | | | | | | | |
| Snack 2 | | | | | | | |
| Snack 3 | | | | | | | |
| Party | | | | | | | |

## Food list

| Vegetables | Grain | Meat |
|---|---|---|
| ☐ Almond | ☐ Adzuki Beans | ☐ Fish |
| ☐ Cabbage | ☐ Barley | ☐ Goat |
| ☐ Carrot | ☐ Black Bean | ☐ Pork |
| ☐ Boccoli | ☐ Brown Rice | ☐ Beef |
| ☐ Garlic | ☐ Buckwheat | ☐ Lamb |
| ☐ Licorice | ☐ Job'sTears, Adlay | ☐ Chicken |
| ☐ Onion | ☐ Millet | ☐ _____ |
| ☐ Spinach | ☐ Mung Beans | ☐ _____ |
| ☐ Sweet potato | ☐ Sesame | ☐ _____ |
| ☐ Tomato | ☐ Sorghum | |
| ☐ _____ | ☐ _____ | |
| ☐ _____ | ☐ _____ | |
| ☐ _____ | ☐ _____ | |

Note:............................................................................................
..........................................................................................
........................................................................................

No........ Date........../..........

| | M | T | W | TH | F | S | S |
|---|---|---|---|---|---|---|---|
| Drink Wather | | | | | | | |
| Breakfast | | | | | | | |
| Lunch | | | | | | | |
| Diner | | | | | | | |
| **Sleep** | | | | | | | |
| **Active** | | | | | | | |
| Snack 1 | | | | | | | |
| **Snack 2** | | | | | | | |
| **Snack 3** | | | | | | | |
| **Party** | | | | | | | |

## Food list

| Vegetables | Grain | Meat |
|---|---|---|
| ☐ Almond | ☐ Adzuki Beans | ☐ Fish |
| ☐ Cabbage | ☐ Barley | ☐ Goat |
| ☐ Carrot | ☐ Black Bean | ☐ Pork |
| ☐ Boccoli | ☐ Brown Rice | ☐ Beef |
| ☐ Garlic | ☐ Buckwheat | ☐ Lamb |
| ☐ Licorice | ☐ Job'sTears, Adlay | ☐ Chicken |
| ☐ Onion | ☐ Millet | ☐ _____ |
| ☐ Spinach | ☐ Mung Beans | ☐ _____ |
| ☐ Sweet potato | ☐ Sesame | ☐ _____ |
| ☐ Tomato | ☐ Sorghum | |
| ☐ _____ | ☐ _____ | |
| ☐ _____ | ☐ _____ | |
| ☐ _____ | ☐ _____ | |

Note:.................................................................................................
.................................................................................................
.................................................................................................

No........ Date........../..........

| | M | T | W | TH | F | S | S |
|---|---|---|---|---|---|---|---|
| Drink Wather | | | | | | | |
| Breakfast | | | | | | | |
| Lunch | | | | | | | |
| Diner | | | | | | | |
| **Sleep** | | | | | | | |
| **Active** | | | | | | | |
| Snack 1 | | | | | | | |
| **Snack 2** | | | | | | | |
| **Snack 3** | | | | | | | |
| **Party** | | | | | | | |

## Food list

| Vegetables | Grain | Meat |
|---|---|---|
| ☐ Almond | ☐ Adzuki Beans | ☐ Fish |
| ☐ Cabbage | ☐ Barley | ☐ Goat |
| ☐ Carrot | ☐ Black Bean | ☐ Pork |
| ☐ Boccoli | ☐ Brown Rice | ☐ Beef |
| ☐ Garlic | ☐ Buckwheat | ☐ Lamb |
| ☐ Licorice | ☐ Job'sTears, Adlay | ☐ Chicken |
| ☐ Onion | ☐ Millet | ☐ _____ |
| ☐ Spinach | ☐ Mung Beans | ☐ _____ |
| ☐ Sweet potato | ☐ Sesame | ☐ _____ |
| ☐ Tomato | ☐ Sorghum | |
| ☐ _____ | ☐ _____ | |
| ☐ _____ | ☐ _____ | |
| ☐ _____ | ☐ _____ | |

Note:...................................................................................................
........................................................................................................
........................................................................................

No........ Date........../..........

| | M | T | W | TH | F | S | S |
|---|---|---|---|---|---|---|---|
| Drink Wather | | | | | | | |
| Breakfast | | | | | | | |
| Lunch | | | | | | | |
| Diner | | | | | | | |
| **Sleep** | | | | | | | |
| **Active** | | | | | | | |
| Snack 1 | | | | | | | |
| **Snack 2** | | | | | | | |
| **Snack 3** | | | | | | | |
| **Party** | | | | | | | |

## Food list

| Vegetables | Grain | Meat |
|---|---|---|
| ☐ Almond | ☐ Adzuki Beans | ☐ Fish |
| ☐ Cabbage | ☐ Barley | ☐ Goat |
| ☐ Carrot | ☐ Black Bean | ☐ Pork |
| ☐ Boccoli | ☐ Brown Rice | ☐ Beef |
| ☐ Garlic | ☐ Buckwheat | ☐ Lamb |
| ☐ Licorice | ☐ Job'sTears, Adlay | ☐ Chicken |
| ☐ Onion | ☐ Millet | ☐ _____ |
| ☐ Spinach | ☐ Mung Beans | ☐ _____ |
| ☐ Sweet potato | ☐ Sesame | ☐ _____ |
| ☐ Tomato | ☐ Sorghum | |
| ☐ _____ | ☐ _____ | |
| ☐ _____ | ☐ _____ | |
| ☐ _____ | ☐ _____ | |

Note:..............................................................................................
....................................................................................................
....................................................................................................

No........ Date........./..........

| | M | T | W | TH | F | S | S |
|---|---|---|---|---|---|---|---|
| Drink Wather | | | | | | | |
| Breakfast | | | | | | | |
| Lunch | | | | | | | |
| Diner | | | | | | | |
| **Sleep** | | | | | | | |
| **Active** | | | | | | | |
| Snack 1 | | | | | | | |
| **Snack 2** | | | | | | | |
| **Snack 3** | | | | | | | |
| **Party** | | | | | | | |

## Food list

| Vegetables | Grain | Meat |
|---|---|---|
| ☐ Almond | ☐ Adzuki Beans | ☐ Fish |
| ☐ Cabbage | ☐ Barley | ☐ Goat |
| ☐ Carrot | ☐ Black Bean | ☐ Pork |
| ☐ Boccoli | ☐ Brown Rice | ☐ Beef |
| ☐ Garlic | ☐ Buckwheat | ☐ Lamb |
| ☐ Licorice | ☐ Job'sTears, Adlay | ☐ Chicken |
| ☐ Onion | ☐ Millet | ☐ _____ |
| ☐ Spinach | ☐ Mung Beans | ☐ _____ |
| ☐ Sweet potato | ☐ Sesame | ☐ _____ |
| ☐ Tomato | ☐ Sorghum | |
| ☐ _____ | ☐ _____ | |
| ☐ _____ | ☐ _____ | |
| ☐ _____ | ☐ _____ | |

Note:...........................................................................................
............................................................................................
............................................................................................

No........ Date........../..........

| | M | T | W | TH | F | S | S |
|---|---|---|---|---|---|---|---|
| Drink Wather | | | | | | | |
| Breakfast | | | | | | | |
| Lunch | | | | | | | |
| Diner | | | | | | | |
| **Sleep** | | | | | | | |
| **Active** | | | | | | | |
| Snack 1 | | | | | | | |
| **Snack 2** | | | | | | | |
| **Snack 3** | | | | | | | |
| **Party** | | | | | | | |

## Food list

| Vegetables | Grain | Meat |
|---|---|---|
| ☐ Almond | ☐ Adzuki Beans | ☐ Fish |
| ☐ Cabbage | ☐ Barley | ☐ Goat |
| ☐ Carrot | ☐ Black Bean | ☐ Pork |
| ☐ Boccoli | ☐ Brown Rice | ☐ Beef |
| ☐ Garlic | ☐ Buckwheat | ☐ Lamb |
| ☐ Licorice | ☐ Job'sTears, Adlay | ☐ Chicken |
| ☐ Onion | ☐ Millet | ☐ _____ |
| ☐ Spinach | ☐ Mung Beans | ☐ _____ |
| ☐ Sweet potato | ☐ Sesame | ☐ _____ |
| ☐ Tomato | ☐ Sorghum | |
| ☐ _____ | ☐ _____ | |
| ☐ _____ | ☐ _____ | |
| ☐ _____ | ☐ _____ | |

Note:........................................................................................
........................................................................................
........................................................................................

No........ Date........../..........

| | M | T | W | TH | F | S | S |
|---|---|---|---|---|---|---|---|
| Drink Wather | | | | | | | |
| Breakfast | | | | | | | |
| Lunch | | | | | | | |
| Diner | | | | | | | |
| **Sleep** | | | | | | | |
| **Active** | | | | | | | |
| Snack 1 | | | | | | | |
| **Snack 2** | | | | | | | |
| **Snack 3** | | | | | | | |
| **Party** | | | | | | | |

## Food list

| Vegetables | Grain | Meat |
|---|---|---|
| ☐ Almond | ☐ Adzuki Beans | ☐ Fish |
| ☐ Cabbage | ☐ Barley | ☐ Goat |
| ☐ Carrot | ☐ Black Bean | ☐ Pork |
| ☐ Boccoli | ☐ Brown Rice | ☐ Beef |
| ☐ Garlic | ☐ Buckwheat | ☐ Lamb |
| ☐ Licorice | ☐ Job'sTears, Adlay | ☐ Chicken |
| ☐ Onion | ☐ Millet | ☐ _____ |
| ☐ Spinach | ☐ Mung Beans | ☐ _____ |
| ☐ Sweet potato | ☐ Sesame | ☐ _____ |
| ☐ Tomato | ☐ Sorghum | |
| ☐ _____ | ☐ _____ | |
| ☐ _____ | ☐ _____ | |
| ☐ _____ | ☐ _____ | |

Note:...........................................................................................
..................................................................................................
..................................................................................................

No........ Date........../..........

| | M | T | W | TH | F | S | S |
|---|---|---|---|---|---|---|---|
| Drink Wather | | | | | | | |
| Breakfast | | | | | | | |
| Lunch | | | | | | | |
| Diner | | | | | | | |
| **Sleep** | | | | | | | |
| **Active** | | | | | | | |
| Snack 1 | | | | | | | |
| **Snack 2** | | | | | | | |
| **Snack 3** | | | | | | | |
| **Party** | | | | | | | |

## Food list

| Vegetables | Grain | Meat |
|---|---|---|
| ☐ Almond | ☐ Adzuki Beans | ☐ Fish |
| ☐ Cabbage | ☐ Barley | ☐ Goat |
| ☐ Carrot | ☐ Black Bean | ☐ Pork |
| ☐ Boccoli | ☐ Brown Rice | ☐ Beef |
| ☐ Garlic | ☐ Buckwheat | ☐ Lamb |
| ☐ Licorice | ☐ Job'sTears, Adlay | ☐ Chicken |
| ☐ Onion | ☐ Millet, | ☐ _____ |
| ☐ Spinach | ☐ Mung Beans | ☐ _____ |
| ☐ Sweet potato | ☐ Sesame | ☐ _____ |
| ☐ Tomato | ☐ Sorghum | |
| ☐ _____ | ☐ _____ | |
| ☐ _____ | ☐ _____ | |
| ☐ _____ | ☐ _____ | |

Note:....................................................................................................
....................................................................................................
....................................................................................................

No........ Date........../..........

| | M | T | W | TH | F | S | S |
|---|---|---|---|---|---|---|---|
| Drink Wather | | | | | | | |
| Breakfast | | | | | | | |
| Lunch | | | | | | | |
| Diner | | | | | | | |
| **Sleep** | | | | | | | |
| **Active** | | | | | | | |
| Snack 1 | | | | | | | |
| **Snack 2** | | | | | | | |
| **Snack 3** | | | | | | | |
| **Party** | | | | | | | |

## Food list

| Vegetables | Grain | Meat |
|---|---|---|
| ☐ Almond | ☐ Adzuki Beans | ☐ Fish |
| ☐ Cabbage | ☐ Barley | ☐ Goat |
| ☐ Carrot | ☐ Black Bean | ☐ Pork |
| ☐ Boccoli | ☐ Brown Rice | ☐ Beef |
| ☐ Garlic | ☐ Buckwheat | ☐ Lamb |
| ☐ Licorice | ☐ Job'sTears, Adlay | ☐ Chicken |
| ☐ Onion | ☐ Millet | ☐ _____ |
| ☐ Spinach | ☐ Mung Beans | ☐ _____ |
| ☐ Sweet potato | ☐ Sesame | ☐ _____ |
| ☐ Tomato | ☐ Sorghum | |
| ☐ _____ | ☐ _____ | |
| ☐ _____ | ☐ _____ | |
| ☐ _____ | ☐ _____ | |

Note:................................................................................
................................................................................
................................................................................

No........ Date........../..........

| | M | T | W | TH | F | S | S |
|---|---|---|---|---|---|---|---|
| Drink Wather | | | | | | | |
| Breakfast | | | | | | | |
| Lunch | | | | | | | |
| Diner | | | | | | | |
| **Sleep** | | | | | | | |
| **Active** | | | | | | | |
| Snack 1 | | | | | | | |
| **Snack 2** | | | | | | | |
| **Snack 3** | | | | | | | |
| **Party** | | | | | | | |

## Food List

| Vegetables | Grain | Meat |
|---|---|---|
| ☐ Almond | ☐ Adzuki Beans | ☐ Fish |
| ☐ Cabbage | ☐ Barley | ☐ Goat |
| ☐ Carrot | ☐ Black Bean | ☐ Pork |
| ☐ Boccoli | ☐ Brown Rice | ☐ Beef |
| ☐ Garlic | ☐ Buckwheat | ☐ Lamb |
| ☐ Licorice | ☐ Job'sTears, Adlay | ☐ Chicken |
| ☐ Onion | ☐ Millet | ☐ _____ |
| ☐ Spinach | ☐ Mung Beans | ☐ _____ |
| ☐ Sweet potato | ☐ Sesame | ☐ _____ |
| ☐ Tomato | ☐ Sorghum | |
| ☐ _____ | ☐ _____ | |
| ☐ _____ | ☐ _____ | |
| ☐ _____ | ☐ _____ | |

Note:.............................................................................................
.............................................................................................
.............................................................................................

No........ Date........../..........

| | M | T | W | TH | F | S | S |
|---|---|---|---|---|---|---|---|
| Drink Wather | | | | | | | |
| Breakfast | | | | | | | |
| Lunch | | | | | | | |
| Diner | | | | | | | |
| **Sleep** | | | | | | | |
| **Active** | | | | | | | |
| Snack 1 | | | | | | | |
| **Snack 2** | | | | | | | |
| **Snack 3** | | | | | | | |
| **Party** | | | | | | | |

## Food list

| **Vegetables** | **Grain** | **Meat** |
|---|---|---|
| ☐ Almond | ☐ Adzuki Beans | ☐ Fish |
| ☐ Cabbage | ☐ Barley | ☐ Goat |
| ☐ Carrot | ☐ Black Bean | ☐ Pork |
| ☐ Boccoli | ☐ Brown Rice | ☐ Beef |
| ☐ Garlic | ☐ Buckwheat | ☐ Lamb |
| ☐ Licorice | ☐ Job'sTears, Adlay | ☐ Chicken |
| ☐ Onion | ☐ Millet | ☐ _____ |
| ☐ Spinach | ☐ Mung Beans | ☐ _____ |
| ☐ Sweet potato | ☐ Sesame | ☐ _____ |
| ☐ Tomato | ☐ Sorghum | |
| ☐ _____ | ☐ _____ | |
| ☐ _____ | ☐ _____ | |
| ☐ _____ | ☐ _____ | |

Note:........................................................................................................
...............................................................................................................
...............................................................................................................

No........ Date........../..........

| | M | T | W | TH | F | S | S |
|---|---|---|---|---|---|---|---|
| Drink Wather | | | | | | | |
| Breakfast | | | | | | | |
| Lunch | | | | | | | |
| Diner | | | | | | | |
| **Sleep** | | | | | | | |
| **Active** | | | | | | | |
| Snack 1 | | | | | | | |
| **Snack 2** | | | | | | | |
| **Snack 3** | | | | | | | |
| **Party** | | | | | | | |

## Food List

| Vegetables | Grain | Meat |
|---|---|---|
| ☐ Almond | ☐ Adzuki Beans | ☐ Fish |
| ☐ Cabbage | ☐ Barley | ☐ Goat |
| ☐ Carrot | ☐ Black Bean | ☐ Pork |
| ☐ Boccoli | ☐ Brown Rice | ☐ Beef |
| ☐ Garlic | ☐ Buckwheat | ☐ Lamb |
| ☐ Licorice | ☐ Job'sTears, Adlay | ☐ Chicken |
| ☐ Onion | ☐ Millet | ☐ _____ |
| ☐ Spinach | ☐ Mung Beans | ☐ _____ |
| ☐ Sweet potato | ☐ Sesame | ☐ _____ |
| ☐ Tomato | ☐ Sorghum | |
| ☐ _____ | ☐ _____ | |
| ☐ _____ | ☐ _____ | |
| ☐ _____ | ☐ _____ | |

Note:.............................................................................................
.............................................................................................
.............................................................................................

No........ Date........../..........

| | M | T | W | TH | F | S | S |
|---|---|---|---|---|---|---|---|
| Drink Wather | | | | | | | |
| Breakfast | | | | | | | |
| Lunch | | | | | | | |
| Diner | | | | | | | |
| **Sleep** | | | | | | | |
| **Active** | | | | | | | |
| Snack 1 | | | | | | | |
| **Snack 2** | | | | | | | |
| **Snack 3** | | | | | | | |
| **Party** | | | | | | | |

## Food list

| Vegetables | Grain | Meat |
|---|---|---|
| ☐ Almond | ☐ Adzuki Beans | ☐ Fish |
| ☐ Cabbage | ☐ Barley | ☐ Goat |
| ☐ Carrot | ☐ Black Bean | ☐ Pork |
| ☐ Boccoli | ☐ Brown Rice | ☐ Beef |
| ☐ Garlic | ☐ Buckwheat | ☐ Lamb |
| ☐ Licorice | ☐ Job'sTears, Adlay | ☐ Chicken |
| ☐ Onion | ☐ Millet | ☐ _____ |
| ☐ Spinach | ☐ Mung Beans | ☐ _____ |
| ☐ Sweet potato | ☐ Sesame | ☐ _____ |
| ☐ Tomato | ☐ Sorghum | |
| ☐ _____ | ☐ _____ | |
| ☐ _____ | ☐ _____ | |
| ☐ _____ | ☐ _____ | |

Note:..............................................................................................
..............................................................................................
..............................................................................................

No........ Date........../..........

| | M | T | W | TH | F | S | S |
|---|---|---|---|---|---|---|---|
| Drink Wather | | | | | | | |
| Breakfast | | | | | | | |
| Lunch | | | | | | | |
| Diner | | | | | | | |
| **Sleep** | | | | | | | |
| **Active** | | | | | | | |
| Snack 1 | | | | | | | |
| **Snack 2** | | | | | | | |
| **Snack 3** | | | | | | | |
| **Party** | | | | | | | |

## Food list

| Vegetables | Grain | Meat |
|---|---|---|
| ☐ Almond | ☐ Adzuki Beans | ☐ Fish |
| ☐ Cabbage | ☐ Barley | ☐ Goat |
| ☐ Carrot | ☐ Black Bean | ☐ Pork |
| ☐ Boccoli | ☐ Brown Rice | ☐ Beef |
| ☐ Garlic | ☐ Buckwheat | ☐ Lamb |
| ☐ Licorice | ☐ Job'sTears, Adlay | ☐ Chicken |
| ☐ Onion | ☐ Millet | ☐ _____ |
| ☐ Spinach | ☐ Mung Beans | ☐ _____ |
| ☐ Sweet potato | ☐ Sesame | ☐ _____ |
| ☐ Tomato | ☐ Sorghum | |
| ☐ _____ | ☐ _____ | |
| ☐ _____ | ☐ _____ | |
| ☐ _____ | ☐ _____ | |

Note:.....................................................................................
................................................................................
................................................................................

No........ Date........../..........

| | M | T | W | TH | F | S | S |
|---|---|---|---|---|---|---|---|
| Drink Wather | | | | | | | |
| Breakfast | | | | | | | |
| Lunch | | | | | | | |
| Diner | | | | | | | |
| **Sleep** | | | | | | | |
| **Active** | | | | | | | |
| Snack 1 | | | | | | | |
| **Snack 2** | | | | | | | |
| **Snack 3** | | | | | | | |
| **Party** | | | | | | | |

## Food list

| Vegetables | Grain | Meat |
|---|---|---|
| ☐ Almond | ☐ Adzuki Beans | ☐ Fish |
| ☐ Cabbage | ☐ Barley | ☐ Goat |
| ☐ Carrot | ☐ Black Bean | ☐ Pork |
| ☐ Boccoli | ☐ Brown Rice | ☐ Beef |
| ☐ Garlic | ☐ Buckwheat | ☐ Lamb |
| ☐ Licorice | ☐ Job'sTears, Adlay | ☐ Chicken |
| ☐ Onion | ☐ Millet | ☐ _____ |
| ☐ Spinach | ☐ Mung Beans | ☐ _____ |
| ☐ Sweet potato | ☐ Sesame | ☐ _____ |
| ☐ Tomato | ☐ Sorghum | |
| ☐ _____ | ☐ _____ | |
| ☐ _____ | ☐ _____ | |
| ☐ _____ | ☐ _____ | |

Note:...............................................................................
.......................................................................................
.......................................................................................

No........ Date........../..........

| | M | T | W | TH | F | S | S |
|---|---|---|---|---|---|---|---|
| Drink Wather | | | | | | | |
| Breakfast | | | | | | | |
| Lunch | | | | | | | |
| Diner | | | | | | | |
| **Sleep** | | | | | | | |
| **Active** | | | | | | | |
| Snack 1 | | | | | | | |
| **Snack 2** | | | | | | | |
| **Snack 3** | | | | | | | |
| **Party** | | | | | | | |

## Food list

| Vegetables | Grain | Meat |
|---|---|---|
| ☐ Almond | ☐ Adzuki Beans | ☐ Fish |
| ☐ Cabbage | ☐ Barley | ☐ Goat |
| ☐ Carrot | ☐ Black Bean | ☐ Pork |
| ☐ Boccoli | ☐ Brown Rice | ☐ Beef |
| ☐ Garlic | ☐ Buckwheat | ☐ Lamb |
| ☐ Licorice | ☐ Job'sTears, Adlay | ☐ Chicken |
| ☐ Onion | ☐ Millet | ☐ _____ |
| ☐ Spinach | ☐ Mung Beans | ☐ _____ |
| ☐ Sweet potato | ☐ Sesame | ☐ _____ |
| ☐ Tomato | ☐ Sorghum | |
| ☐ _____ | ☐ _____ | |
| ☐ _____ | ☐ _____ | |
| ☐ _____ | ☐ _____ | |

Note:......................................................................................................
..........................................................................................................
..........................................................................................................

No........ Date........../..........

| | M | T | W | TH | F | S | S |
|---|---|---|---|---|---|---|---|
| Drink Wather | | | | | | | |
| Breakfast | | | | | | | |
| Lunch | | | | | | | |
| Diner | | | | | | | |
| **Sleep** | | | | | | | |
| **Active** | | | | | | | |
| Snack 1 | | | | | | | |
| **Snack 2** | | | | | | | |
| **Snack 3** | | | | | | | |
| **Party** | | | | | | | |

## Food list

| Vegetables | Grain | Meat |
|---|---|---|
| ☐ Almond | ☐ Adzuki Beans | ☐ Fish |
| ☐ Cabbage | ☐ Barley | ☐ Goat |
| ☐ Carrot | ☐ Black Bean | ☐ Pork |
| ☐ Boccoli | ☐ Brown Rice | ☐ Beef |
| ☐ Garlic | ☐ Buckwheat | ☐ Lamb |
| ☐ Licorice | ☐ Job'sTears, Adlay | ☐ Chicken |
| ☐ Onion | ☐ Millet | ☐ _____ |
| ☐ Spinach | ☐ Mung Beans | ☐ _____ |
| ☐ Sweet potato | ☐ Sesame | ☐ _____ |
| ☐ Tomato | ☐ Sorghum | |
| ☐ _____ | ☐ _____ | |
| ☐ _____ | ☐ _____ | |
| ☐ _____ | ☐ _____ | |

Note:.................................................................................................
...........................................................................................................
...........................................................................................................

No........ Date........../..........

| | M | T | W | TH | F | S | S |
|---|---|---|---|---|---|---|---|
| Drink Wather | | | | | | | |
| Breakfast | | | | | | | |
| Lunch | | | | | | | |
| Diner | | | | | | | |
| **Sleep** | | | | | | | |
| **Active** | | | | | | | |
| Snack 1 | | | | | | | |
| **Snack 2** | | | | | | | |
| **Snack 3** | | | | | | | |
| **Party** | | | | | | | |

## Food List

| Vegetables | Grain | Meat |
|---|---|---|
| ☐ Almond | ☐ Adzuki Beans | ☐ Fish |
| ☐ Cabbage | ☐ Barley | ☐ Goat |
| ☐ Carrot | ☐ Black Bean | ☐ Pork |
| ☐ Boccoli | ☐ Brown Rice | ☐ Beef |
| ☐ Garlic | ☐ Buckwheat | ☐ Lamb |
| ☐ Licorice | ☐ Job'sTears, Adlay | ☐ Chicken |
| ☐ Onion | ☐ Millet | ☐ _____ |
| ☐ Spinach | ☐ Mung Beans | ☐ _____ |
| ☐ Sweet potato | ☐ Sesame | ☐ _____ |
| ☐ Tomato | ☐ Sorghum | |
| ☐ _____ | ☐ _____ | |
| ☐ _____ | ☐ _____ | |
| ☐ _____ | ☐ _____ | |

Note:.................................................................................................
..........................................................................................................
..........................................................................................................

No........ Date........../..........

| | M | T | W | TH | F | S | S |
|---|---|---|---|---|---|---|---|
| Drink Wather | | | | | | | |
| Breakfast | | | | | | | |
| Lunch | | | | | | | |
| Diner | | | | | | | |
| **Sleep** | | | | | | | |
| **Active** | | | | | | | |
| Snack 1 | | | | | | | |
| **Snack 2** | | | | | | | |
| **Snack 3** | | | | | | | |
| **Party** | | | | | | | |

## Food List

| Vegetables | Grain | Meat |
|---|---|---|
| ☐ Almond | ☐ Adzuki Beans | ☐ Fish |
| ☐ Cabbage | ☐ Barley | ☐ Goat |
| ☐ Carrot | ☐ Black Bean | ☐ Pork |
| ☐ Boccoli | ☐ Brown Rice | ☐ Beef |
| ☐ Garlic | ☐ Buckwheat | ☐ Lamb |
| ☐ Licorice | ☐ Job'sTears, Adlay | ☐ Chicken |
| ☐ Onion | ☐ Millet | ☐ _____ |
| ☐ Spinach | ☐ Mung Beans | ☐ _____ |
| ☐ Sweet potato | ☐ Sesame | ☐ _____ |
| ☐ Tomato | ☐ Sorghum | |
| ☐ _____ | ☐ _____ | |
| ☐ _____ | ☐ _____ | |
| ☐ _____ | ☐ _____ | |

Note:................................................................................................
................................................................................................
................................................................................................

No........ Date........../..........

| | M | T | W | TH | F | S | S |
|---|---|---|---|---|---|---|---|
| Drink Wather | | | | | | | |
| Breakfast | | | | | | | |
| Lunch | | | | | | | |
| Diner | | | | | | | |
| **Sleep** | | | | | | | |
| **Active** | | | | | | | |
| Snack 1 | | | | | | | |
| **Snack 2** | | | | | | | |
| **Snack 3** | | | | | | | |
| **Party** | | | | | | | |

## Food list

| Vegetables | Grain | Meat |
|---|---|---|
| ☐ Almond | ☐ Adzuki Beans | ☐ Fish |
| ☐ Cabbage | ☐ Barley | ☐ Goat |
| ☐ Carrot | ☐ Black Bean | ☐ Pork |
| ☐ Boccoli | ☐ Brown Rice | ☐ Beef |
| ☐ Garlic | ☐ Buckwheat | ☐ Lamb |
| ☐ Licorice | ☐ Job'sTears, Adlay | ☐ Chicken |
| ☐ Onion | ☐ Millet | ☐ _____ |
| ☐ Spinach | ☐ Mung Beans | ☐ _____ |
| ☐ Sweet potato | ☐ Sesame | ☐ _____ |
| ☐ Tomato | ☐ Sorghum | |
| ☐ _____ | ☐ _____ | |
| ☐ _____ | ☐ _____ | |
| ☐ _____ | ☐ _____ | |

Note:...........................................................................................
..................................................................................................
..................................................................................................

No........ Date........../..........

| | M | T | W | TH | F | S | S |
|---|---|---|---|---|---|---|---|
| Drink Wather | | | | | | | |
| Breakfast | | | | | | | |
| Lunch | | | | | | | |
| Diner | | | | | | | |
| **Sleep** | | | | | | | |
| **Active** | | | | | | | |
| Snack 1 | | | | | | | |
| **Snack 2** | | | | | | | |
| **Snack 3** | | | | | | | |
| **Party** | | | | | | | |

## Food list

| Vegetables | Grain | Meat |
|---|---|---|
| ☐ Almond | ☐ Adzuki Beans | ☐ Fish |
| ☐ Cabbage | ☐ Barley | ☐ Goat |
| ☐ Carrot | ☐ Black Bean | ☐ Pork |
| ☐ Boccoli | ☐ Brown Rice | ☐ Beef |
| ☐ Garlic | ☐ Buckwheat | ☐ Lamb |
| ☐ Licorice | ☐ Job'sTears, Adlay | ☐ Chicken |
| ☐ Onion | ☐ Millet | ☐ _____ |
| ☐ Spinach | ☐ Mung Beans | ☐ _____ |
| ☐ Sweet potato | ☐ Sesame | ☐ _____ |
| ☐ Tomato | ☐ Sorghum | |
| ☐ _____ | ☐ _____ | |
| ☐ _____ | ☐ _____ | |
| ☐ _____ | ☐ _____ | |

Note:.......................................................................................................
...............................................................................................................
...............................................................................................................

No........ Date........../..........

| | M | T | W | TH | F | S | S |
|---|---|---|---|---|---|---|---|
| Drink Wather | | | | | | | |
| Breakfast | | | | | | | |
| Lunch | | | | | | | |
| Diner | | | | | | | |
| **Sleep** | | | | | | | |
| **Active** | | | | | | | |
| Snack 1 | | | | | | | |
| **Snack 2** | | | | | | | |
| **Snack 3** | | | | | | | |
| **Party** | | | | | | | |

## Food list

| Vegetables | Grain | Meat |
|---|---|---|
| ☐ Almond | ☐ Adzuki Beans | ☐ Fish |
| ☐ Cabbage | ☐ Barley | ☐ Goat |
| ☐ Carrot | ☐ Black Bean | ☐ Pork |
| ☐ Boccoli | ☐ Brown Rice | ☐ Beef |
| ☐ Garlic | ☐ Buckwheat | ☐ Lamb |
| ☐ Licorice | ☐ Job'sTears, Adlay | ☐ Chicken |
| ☐ Onion | ☐ Millet | ☐ _____ |
| ☐ Spinach | ☐ Mung Beans | ☐ _____ |
| ☐ Sweet potato | ☐ Sesame | ☐ _____ |
| ☐ Tomato | ☐ Sorghum | |
| ☐ _____ | ☐ _____ | |
| ☐ _____ | ☐ _____ | |
| ☐ _____ | ☐ _____ | |

Note:................................................................................
.........................................................................................
.........................................................................................

No........ Date........../..........

| | M | T | W | TH | F | S | S |
|---|---|---|---|---|---|---|---|
| Drink Wather | | | | | | | |
| Breakfast | | | | | | | |
| Lunch | | | | | | | |
| Diner | | | | | | | |
| **Sleep** | | | | | | | |
| **Active** | | | | | | | |
| Snack 1 | | | | | | | |
| **Snack 2** | | | | | | | |
| **Snack 3** | | | | | | | |
| Party | | | | | | | |

## Food list

| Vegetables | Grain | Meat |
|---|---|---|
| ☐ Almond | ☐ Adzuki Beans | ☐ Fish |
| ☐ Cabbage | ☐ Barley | ☐ Goat |
| ☐ Carrot | ☐ Black Bean | ☐ Pork |
| ☐ Boccoli | ☐ Brown Rice | ☐ Beef |
| ☐ Garlic | ☐ Buckwheat | ☐ Lamb |
| ☐ Licorice | ☐ Job'sTears, Adlay | ☐ Chicken |
| ☐ Onion | ☐ Millet | ☐ _____ |
| ☐ Spinach | ☐ Mung Beans | ☐ _____ |
| ☐ Sweet potato | ☐ Sesame | ☐ _____ |
| ☐ Tomato | ☐ Sorghum | |
| ☐ _____ | ☐ _____ | |
| ☐ _____ | ☐ _____ | |
| ☐ _____ | ☐ _____ | |

Note:................................................................................................
................................................................................................
................................................................................................

No........ Date........../..........

| | M | T | W | TH | F | S | S |
|---|---|---|---|---|---|---|---|
| Drink Wather | | | | | | | |
| Breakfast | | | | | | | |
| Lunch | | | | | | | |
| Diner | | | | | | | |
| **Sleep** | | | | | | | |
| **Active** | | | | | | | |
| Snack 1 | | | | | | | |
| **Snack 2** | | | | | | | |
| **Snack 3** | | | | | | | |
| **Party** | | | | | | | |

## Food List

| Vegetables | Grain | Meat |
|---|---|---|
| ☐ Almond | ☐ Adzuki Beans | ☐ Fish |
| ☐ Cabbage | ☐ Barley | ☐ Goat |
| ☐ Carrot | ☐ Black Bean | ☐ Pork |
| ☐ Boccoli | ☐ Brown Rice | ☐ Beef |
| ☐ Garlic | ☐ Buckwheat | ☐ Lamb |
| ☐ Licorice | ☐ Job'sTears, Adlay | ☐ Chicken |
| ☐ Onion | ☐ Millet | ☐ _____ |
| ☐ Spinach | ☐ Mung Beans | ☐ _____ |
| ☐ Sweet potato | ☐ Sesame | ☐ _____ |
| ☐ Tomato | ☐ Sorghum | |
| ☐ _____ | ☐ _____ | |
| ☐ _____ | ☐ _____ | |
| ☐ _____ | ☐ _____ | |

Note:....................................................................................
..............................................................................................
..............................................................................................

No........ Date........../..........

| | M | T | W | TH | F | S | S |
|---|---|---|---|---|---|---|---|
| Drink Wather | | | | | | | |
| Breakfast | | | | | | | |
| Lunch | | | | | | | |
| Diner | | | | | | | |
| **Sleep** | | | | | | | |
| **Active** | | | | | | | |
| Snack 1 | | | | | | | |
| **Snack 2** | | | | | | | |
| **Snack 3** | | | | | | | |
| **Party** | | | | | | | |

## Food list

| Vegetables | Grain | Meat |
|---|---|---|
| ☐ Almond | ☐ Adzuki Beans | ☐ Fish |
| ☐ Cabbage | ☐ Barley | ☐ Goat |
| ☐ Carrot | ☐ Black Bean | ☐ Pork |
| ☐ Boccoli | ☐ Brown Rice | ☐ Beef |
| ☐ Garlic | ☐ Buckwheat | ☐ Lamb |
| ☐ Licorice | ☐ Job'sTears, Adlay | ☐ Chicken |
| ☐ Onion | ☐ Millet | ☐ _____ |
| ☐ Spinach | ☐ Mung Beans | ☐ _____ |
| ☐ Sweet potato | ☐ Sesame | ☐ _____ |
| ☐ Tomato | ☐ Sorghum | |
| ☐ _____ | ☐ _____ | |
| ☐ _____ | ☐ _____ | |
| ☐ _____ | ☐ _____ | |

Note:...............................................................................
........................................................................................
........................................................................................

No........ Date........../..........

| | M | T | W | TH | F | S | S |
|---|---|---|---|---|---|---|---|
| Drink Wather | | | | | | | |
| Breakfast | | | | | | | |
| Lunch | | | | | | | |
| Diner | | | | | | | |
| **Sleep** | | | | | | | |
| **Active** | | | | | | | |
| Snack 1 | | | | | | | |
| **Snack 2** | | | | | | | |
| **Snack 3** | | | | | | | |
| **Party** | | | | | | | |

## Food list

| Vegetables | Grain | Meat |
|---|---|---|
| ☐ Almond | ☐ Adzuki Beans | ☐ Fish |
| ☐ Cabbage | ☐ Barley | ☐ Goat |
| ☐ Carrot | ☐ Black Bean | ☐ Pork |
| ☐ Boccoli | ☐ Brown Rice | ☐ Beef |
| ☐ Garlic | ☐ Buckwheat | ☐ Lamb |
| ☐ Licorice | ☐ Job'sTears, Adlay | ☐ Chicken |
| ☐ Onion | ☐ Millet | ☐ _____ |
| ☐ Spinach | ☐ Mung Beans | ☐ _____ |
| ☐ Sweet potato | ☐ Sesame | ☐ _____ |
| ☐ Tomato | ☐ Sorghum | |
| ☐ _____ | ☐ _____ | |
| ☐ _____ | ☐ _____ | |
| ☐ _____ | ☐ _____ | |

Note:.................................................................................................
.................................................................................................
.................................................................................................

No........ Date........../..........

| | M | T | W | TH | F | S | S |
|---|---|---|---|---|---|---|---|
| Drink Wather | | | | | | | |
| Breakfast | | | | | | | |
| Lunch | | | | | | | |
| Diner | | | | | | | |
| **Sleep** | | | | | | | |
| **Active** | | | | | | | |
| Snack 1 | | | | | | | |
| **Snack 2** | | | | | | | |
| **Snack 3** | | | | | | | |
| **Party** | | | | | | | |

## Food list

| Vegetables | Grain | Meat |
|---|---|---|
| ☐ Almond | ☐ Adzuki Beans | ☐ Fish |
| ☐ Cabbage | ☐ Barley | ☐ Goat |
| ☐ Carrot | ☐ Black Bean | ☐ Pork |
| ☐ Boccoli | ☐ Brown Rice | ☐ Beef |
| ☐ Garlic | ☐ Buckwheat | ☐ Lamb |
| ☐ Licorice | ☐ Job'sTears, Adlay | ☐ Chicken |
| ☐ Onion | ☐ Millet | ☐ _____ |
| ☐ Spinach | ☐ Mung Beans | ☐ _____ |
| ☐ Sweet potato | ☐ Sesame | ☐ _____ |
| ☐ Tomato | ☐ Sorghum | |
| ☐ _____ | ☐ _____ | |
| ☐ _____ | ☐ _____ | |
| ☐ _____ | ☐ _____ | |

Note:.......................................................................................................
............................................................................................................
............................................................................................................

No........ Date........../..........

| | M | T | W | TH | F | S | S |
|---|---|---|---|---|---|---|---|
| Drink Wather | | | | | | | |
| Breakfast | | | | | | | |
| Lunch | | | | | | | |
| Diner | | | | | | | |
| **Sleep** | | | | | | | |
| **Active** | | | | | | | |
| Snack 1 | | | | | | | |
| **Snack 2** | | | | | | | |
| **Snack 3** | | | | | | | |
| **Party** | | | | | | | |

## Food list

| Vegetables | Grain | Meat |
|---|---|---|
| ☐ Almond | ☐ Adzuki Beans | ☐ Fish |
| ☐ Cabbage | ☐ Barley | ☐ Goat |
| ☐ Carrot | ☐ Black Bean | ☐ Pork |
| ☐ Boccoli | ☐ Brown Rice | ☐ Beef |
| ☐ Garlic | ☐ Buckwheat | ☐ Lamb |
| ☐ Licorice | ☐ Job'sTears, Adlay | ☐ Chicken |
| ☐ Onion | ☐ Millet | ☐ _____ |
| ☐ Spinach | ☐ Mung Beans | ☐ _____ |
| ☐ Sweet potato | ☐ Sesame | ☐ _____ |
| ☐ Tomato | ☐ Sorghum | |
| ☐ _____ | ☐ _____ | |
| ☐ _____ | ☐ _____ | |
| ☐ _____ | ☐ _____ | |

Note:.............................................................................................................
..........................................................................................................................
..........................................................................................................................

No........ Date........../..........

| | M | T | W | TH | F | S | S |
|---|---|---|---|---|---|---|---|
| Drink Wather | | | | | | | |
| Breakfast | | | | | | | |
| Lunch | | | | | | | |
| Diner | | | | | | | |
| **Sleep** | | | | | | | |
| **Active** | | | | | | | |
| Snack 1 | | | | | | | |
| **Snack 2** | | | | | | | |
| **Snack 3** | | | | | | | |
| **Party** | | | | | | | |

## Food list

| Vegetables | Grain | Meat |
|---|---|---|
| ☐ Almond | ☐ Adzuki Beans | ☐ Fish |
| ☐ Cabbage | ☐ Barley | ☐ Goat |
| ☐ Carrot | ☐ Black Bean | ☐ Pork |
| ☐ Boccoli | ☐ Brown Rice | ☐ Beef |
| ☐ Garlic | ☐ Buckwheat | ☐ Lamb |
| ☐ Licorice | ☐ Job'sTears, Adlay | ☐ Chicken |
| ☐ Onion | ☐ Millet | ☐ _____ |
| ☐ Spinach | ☐ Mung Beans | ☐ _____ |
| ☐ Sweet potato | ☐ Sesame | ☐ _____ |
| ☐ Tomato | ☐ Sorghum | |
| ☐ _____ | ☐ _____ | |
| ☐ _____ | ☐ _____ | |
| ☐ _____ | ☐ _____ | |

Note:.............................................................................................
............................................................................................................
............................................................................................................

How can you be sucessful in Healthy data?

........................................................................................
........................................................................................
........................................................................................
........................................................................................
........................................................................................
........................................................................................
........................................................................................
........................................................................................
........................................................................................
........................................................................................
........................................................................................
........................................................................................
........................................................................................
........................................................................................
........................................................................................
........................................................................................
........................................................................................
........................................................................................
........................................................................................
........................................................................................
........................................................................................
........................................................................................
........................................................................................
........................................................................................
........................................................................................
........................................................................................
........................................................................................
........................................................................................
........................................................................................
........................................................................................
........................................................................................
........................................................................................
........................................................................................
........................................................................................
........................................................................................
........................................................................................
........................................................................................
........................................................................................